BODY WEIGHT WORKOUTS FOR SENIORS

A COMPLETE GUIDE TO AGE-DEFYING FITNESS

RICHARD E. MARSHALL

GET ACCESS TO MY MORE FITNESS BOOKS

CONTENTS:

INTRODUCTION

Seniors benefit greatly from bodyweight exercises since they are low impact and adaptable to all levels of fitness. They may be performed anytime, anyplace, and without the need for any equipment. Additionally, bodyweight exercises are a great way to increase strength, enhance flexibility and balance, and lower the chance of falling.

Bodyweight exercises let elders do resistance training without the extra stress of traditional weightlifting, which can damage muscles and joints. Bodyweight exercises are a great way to promote functional strength and lower the chance of injury in later life since they resemble everyday actions. These senior-specific workouts, which range from mild squats to seated leg lifts, provide a well-rounded approach to fitness.

Bodyweight Excrcises Benefits for Seniors

Exercises using bodyweight are very beneficial outside of the gym. Seniors who use these activities report feeling happier and more mentally healthy. The blood circulation is improved by the rhythmic flow of motions, which results in heightened energy and vitality. Endorphins, which are commonly referred to be the body's natural mood

enhancers, are released when a person feels good and
hopeful about life

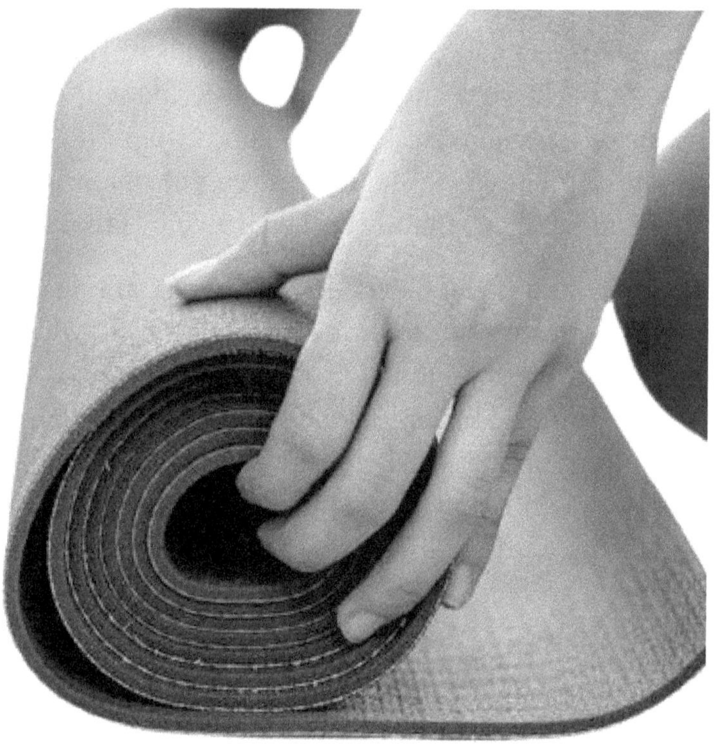

Additionally, bodyweight exercises help elders connect
with others. A supportive community is created when
people who are devoted to their health get together, which
lessens feelings of loneliness and isolation. This social

component turns into a driving factor that helps elders maintain consistency in their exercise regimens and builds enduring relationships.

Strengthening: Seniors who engage in bodyweight exercises can develop and preserve their muscular mass. This is significant since muscle mass declines with age, and a robust muscular system can support seniors' independence and facilitate their performance of everyday tasks.

Enhanced flexibility and balance: Bodyweight exercises can also aid in enhancing flexibility and balance. Seniors should take note of this as it may lower their chance of falling. Maintaining safety and independence requires increasing balance and flexibility, as falls are a major cause of injuries and deaths among the elderly.

Decreased risk of chronic diseases: Exercises using just bodyweight can also help lower the chance of developing long-term conditions like osteoporosis, heart disease, stroke, and type 2 diabetes. One of the greatest methods to enhance general health and lower the risk of chronic illnesses is to exercise, and bodyweight exercises are a quick and efficient way to do it.

Better mental health: Bodyweight exercises are another way to enhance mental well-being. Exercise has been demonstrated to enhance mood and sleep quality while lowering stress, anxiety, and depression. Bodyweight exercises may be a fantastic approach for seniors to enhance their general mental and physical health.

Getting Started with Bodyweight Workouts:

Seniors who want to live a healthier, more active lifestyle can take a powerful step by starting bodyweight exercises. Starting anything new doesn't mean going above and above; instead, it means taking a measured and individualized approach. To assist elders in starting this rewarding fitness journey, below is a road map:

Consultation and Evaluation: Seniors must speak with their healthcare professional prior to starting any exercise program. A complete assessment of one's health situation guarantees that the workouts selected are suitable for one's demands and safe.

Take First Aid and Basics: Start with basic mobility-focused workouts like range-of-motion routines and mild stretches. This builds a strong foundation and gets the body ready for later, more difficult exercises.

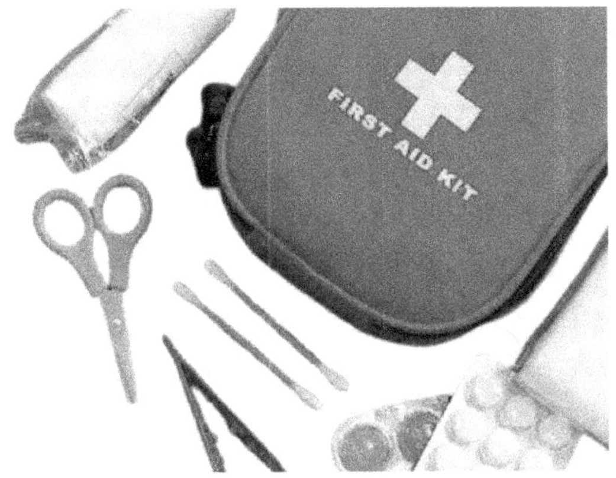

Advance Gradually: Seniors can progressively add more difficult bodyweight exercises as their strength and confidence increase. Adjust the program to suit your comfort level and make any adjustments.

Maintaining consistency is essential for any fitness program to be successful. Seniors should be encouraged to create a regular exercise routine and to progressively increase the length and intensity of their workouts.

Tips for staying motivated and on track

- Maintaining your motivation and focus during your bodyweight exercises is crucial. Here are some pointers:

- Find a workout partner who can assist you in maintaining accountability.
- Make sure your goals are reasonable.
- Follow your development and acknowledge your accomplishments.
- Give yourself a reward for maintaining your exercise schedule.

CHAPTER 1

Senior warm-up exercises

As crucial as a warm-up is to any exercise regimen, older citizens should prioritize it even more. By raising your heart rate, blood flow, and muscle temperature, warming up aids in getting your body ready for physical exertion. It may also assist in lowering your chance of being hurt.

Warm-up sample routine for seniors

Start with 5 to 10 minutes of gentle aerobic exercise, including arm circles, strolling, or place marches.

Dynamic stretches: These are a type of stretch that need motion. They are an effective method of getting your muscles warmed up and ready for activity. Dynamic stretches include, for instance:

- **Arm swings:** Swing your arms in little circles at first, then progressively enlarge them.
- **Leg swings:** Move your legs side to side, back and forth, and forward.
- **Neck rolls:** Roll your head gently from front to back and side to side.
- **Shoulder rolls:** Extend and retract your shoulders.

Static stretches: These are stretches that are held in place for a certain amount of time. They are a useful tool for increasing your range of motion. Static stretches include, for instance:

- Stretch your hamstrings by sitting on the floor and extending your legs in front of you. Stretch toward your toes while maintaining a straight back.
- Stretch your quadriceps by standing behind a chair and placing your hands on the back. Grab your foot with your hand while bending one leg behind you. Bring your heel gently up to your buttocks.
- To stretch your calf, face the wall and place your hands shoulder-height on the wall. Keeping your heel on the ground, take a single-leg step rearward. Till the calf muscle in your rear leg stretches, bend forward.

Cardiovascular Activation: Use low-impact cardiovascular workouts to gradually raise heart rate. Muscles have greater blood flow when you walk quickly or march in place for a short while, which gets them ready for more dynamic actions.

Deep breathing exercises may be included into mindful breathing to help the body and mind become more focused. Breathe in gently through the nose to expand the belly;

exhale through pursed lips to promote relaxation and release tension.

Seniors' cool-down exercises

A warm-up is not as vital as a cool-down. It facilitates your body's recuperation after exertion and transition back to rest. Muscle discomfort can also be lessened by cooling down.

cool-down sample routine for seniors

Start with 5 to 10 minutes of gentle aerobic exercise, including arm circles, strolling, or place marches.

Static stretches: You may include the same static stretches from your warm-up into your cool-down.

Practice deep breathing: Deep breathing techniques can aid in mental and physical relaxation. Take a slow, deep breath through your nose to begin a deep breathing practice. Breathe out slowly through your lips.

Mild Cardiovascular Exercise: After a short period of low-impact cardiovascular exercise, gradually reduce the intensity of your movements. To progressively reduce the pulse rate, this may involve taking a leisurely stroll or marching at a slow speed.

Hydration and Reflection: Stress the need of replenishing fluids after physical activity. Drinking water aids in regaining fluids lost during exercise. Take a minute to reflect as well, praising the session's accomplishments and making plans for better workouts in the future.

warming up and cooling down tips

- Take note of your body. The moment you experience any pain, cease the workout.
- Don't overwork yourself. Exercises for the warm-up and cool-down should be performed at a comfortable tempo.
- Sip a lot of water. Hydration is crucial before, during, and after physical activity.
- Remain dependable. Prior to and following each session, warm up and cool down.

Additional tips

- Put on relaxed attire and comfy shoes.
- Work out in a place with good ventilation.
- Don't work out in extremely cold or hot weather.
- To prevent falls, pay attention to your surroundings and adopt safety measures.

CHAPTER 2

Upper Body Exercises

Push-ups

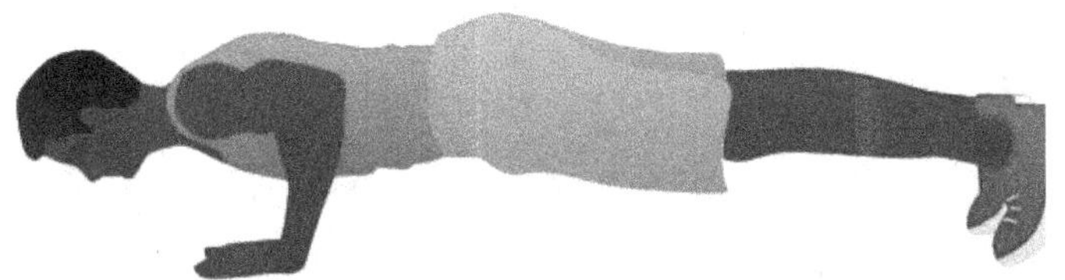

Target area: Chest, triceps, shoulders

Steps:

1. With your hands shoulder-width apart and your body forming a straight line from your head to your heels, start in the plank position.
2. Once your chest contacts the floor, lower your body.
3. Return to the starting position by pushing up.

Reps: 3 sets of 10-12 repetitions

Modifications:

- If you can't perform a full push-up, you can begin by putting your hands on your knees or against a wall.
- To increase or decrease the difficulty of push-ups, you may also utilize a resistance band.

Pull-ups

Target area: Back, biceps, shoulders

Steps:

1. With an overhand hold, slightly wider than shoulder-width apart, grab a pull-up bar.
2. Arrange your arms so that they hang freely from the bar.
3. Raise your chin till it touches the bar.
4. Retrace your steps to the beginning point slowly.

Reps: 3 sets of as many repetitions as possible

Modifications:

- If you are unable to do a full pull-up, you can use a resistance band to assist you.
- You can also use a pull-up assist machine.

Rows

Target area: Back, biceps

Steps:

1. Maintain a straight back and bend at the waist.
2. Hold a pair of dumbbells or a resistance band shoulder-width apart in an overhand grip.
3. Raise the resistance band or dumbbells up to your chest.
4. Return the resistance band or dumbbells to their initial position slowly.

Reps: 3 sets of 10-12 repetitions

Chest press

Target area: Chest, triceps, shoulders

Steps:

1. With your knees bent and your feet flat on the floor, assume a bench position.
2. Holding a pair of dumbbells at chest height, place your hands facing one another.
3. Raise the dumbbells so that your arms are completely stretched.
4. Return the dumbbells to their starting position slowly.

Reps: 3 sets of 10-12 repetitions

Shoulder press

Target area: Shoulders, triceps

Steps:

1. With your back straight and your feet flat on the ground, take a seat on a bench.
2. With your hands pointing front, take a pair of dumbbells and hold them at shoulder height.
3. Raise the dumbbells so that your arms are completely stretched.
4. Return the dumbbells to their starting position slowly.

Reps: 3 sets of 10-12 repetition

Bicep curls

Target area: Biceps

Steps:

1. Holding a pair of dumbbells, stand with your feet shoulder-width apart and your arms at your sides.
2. Keeping your upper arms close to your sides, curl the dumbbells up towards your shoulders.
3. Return the dumbbells to their starting position slowly.

Reps: 3 sets of 10-12 repetitions

Tricep extensions

Target area: Triceps

Steps:

1. Stand with your feet shoulder-width apart and your arms overhead, holding a pair of dumbbells.
2. Bend your elbows and lower the dumbbells behind your head.
3. Straighten your elbows and press the dumbbells back overhead.

Reps: 3 sets of 10-12 repetitions

Lateral raises

Target area: Shoulders

Steps:

1. Holding a pair of dumbbells, stand with your feet shoulder-width apart and your arms at your sides.
2. Until your arms are parallel to the ground, extend them out to the sides.
3. Return your arms to the beginning position slowly.

Reps: 3 sets of 10-12 repetitions

Face pulls

Target area: Shoulders, back

Steps:

1. Use a pull-up bar or other high anchor point to fasten a resistance band.
2. Hold the resistance band's ends shoulder-width apart using an overhand grip.

3. Keeping your elbows up, pull the resistance band in the direction of your face.
4. Return the resistance band to its initial position gradually.

Reps: 3 sets of 10-12 repetitions

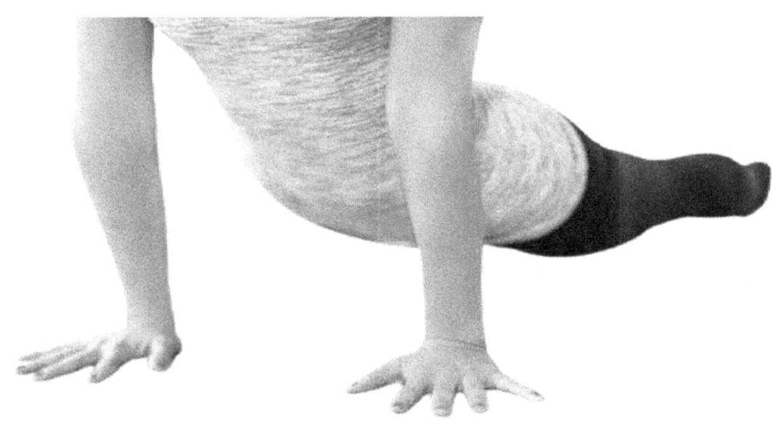

Overhead tricep extensions

Target area: Triceps

Steps:

1. Place your feet shoulder-width apart and grip a pair of dumbbells with your arms raised over your head.
2. Lower the dumbbells behind your head while bending your elbows.
3. Raise your elbows straight and raise the dumbbells back up.

Reps: 3 sets of 10-12 repetitions

CHAPTER 3

Core Exercises

Planks

Target area: Core, abs, back, shoulders

Steps:

1. Start with your forearms on the ground in the push-up position.
2. Keep your body in a straight posture from your head to your heels.
3. Hold the position for as long as possible.

Reps: 3 sets of 30-60 seconds

Modifications:

- Start on your knees if you can't perform a complete plank.
- Alternatively, you might utilize your elbows in place of your forearms.

Crunches

Target area: Abs

Steps:

1. Lying on your back, place your feet flat on the floor and bend your knees.
2. Your hands should be behind your head.
3. With your back on the ground, curl your upper body up towards your knees.
4. Retrace your steps to the starting point slowly.

Reps: 3 sets of 15-20 repetitions

Leg raises

Target area: Lower abs

Steps:

1. Lying on your back, stretch your legs in front of you.
2. Lift your legs gradually until they are parallel to the ground.
3. Slowly bring your legs back to the start position.

Reps: 3 sets of 10-15 repetitions

Russian twists

Target area: Core, obliques

Steps:

1. With your feet flat on the ground and your knees bent, take a seat on the ground.
2. Place a weight plate or medicine ball in front of your chest.
3. Turn your body to one side and lower the weight plate or medicine ball to the floor.
4. Twist back to the initial position and repeat on the other side.

Reps: 3 sets of 10-15 repetitions on each side

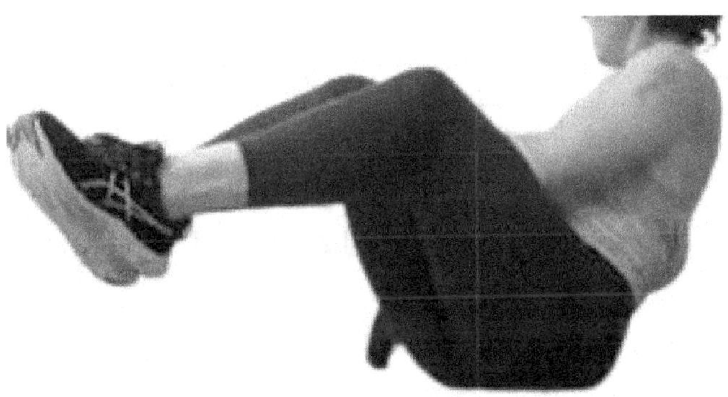

Bird dogs

Target area: Core, back

Steps:

1. With your back straight, begin on your hands and knees.
2. Extend your right arm and left leg out straight.
3. Hold the position for 3 seconds.
4. Go back to where you were before and repeat on the opposite side.

Reps: 3 sets of 10-15 repetitions on each side

Mountain climbers

Target area: Core, abs, shoulders

Steps:

1. With your hands shoulder-width apart and your body forming a straight line from your head to your heels, begin in the plank position.
2. Maintaining an engaged core, bring your right knee forward toward your chest.
3. Step back to the beginning and repeat with your left leg.
4. Maintain the fast leg rotation as much as you can.

Reps: 3 sets of 20-30 repetitions on each leg

Side planks

Target area: Core, obliques

Steps:

1. As you lay on your right side, keep your body in a straight line from your head to your heels by placing your right forearm on the floor.
2. Stack your left and right feet atop each other.
3. Raise your arm to the left above.
4. Hold the position as long as you are able.
5. Continue on the opposite side.

Reps: 3 sets of 30-60 seconds on each side

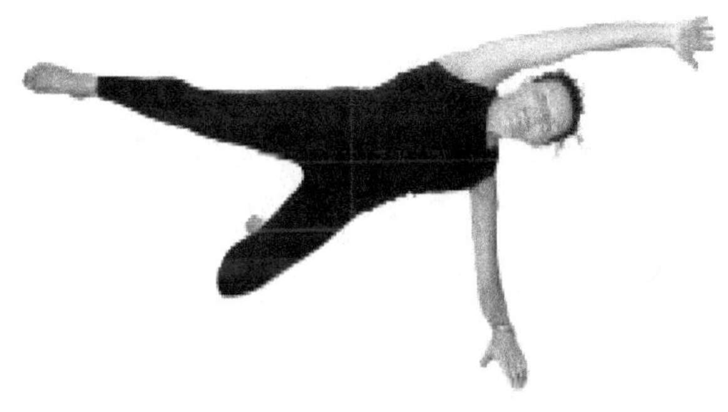

Hollow body hold

Target area: Core, abs

Steps:

1. Place your legs outstretched and your arms aloft while lying on your back.
2. With your back slightly arched, draw your navel toward your spine.
3. Hold the position for as long as possible.

Reps: 3 sets of 30-60 seconds

CHAPTER 4

Squats

Target area: Quadriceps, hamstrings, glutes, calves

Steps:

1. Stand with your feet shoulder-width apart and your toes slightly pointed outward.
2. Bend your knees and lower your body down until your thighs are parallel to the ground.
3. Push back up to the starting position.

Reps: 3 sets of 10-15 repetitions

Modifications:

- If you are unable to do a full squat, you can start by sitting in a chair and standing up.
- You can also use a resistance band to make squats easier or more difficult.

Lunges

Target area: Quadriceps, hamstrings, glutes

Steps:

1. Stand with your feet shoulder-width apart.
2. Step forward with your right leg and lower your body down until both knees are bent at a 90-degree angle.
3. Make sure that your right knee is over your right ankle and your left knee is directly below your left hip.
4. Push back up to the starting position and repeat with your left leg.

Reps: 3 sets of 10-15 repetitions on each leg

Calf raises

Target area: Calves

Steps:

1. Stand with your feet shoulder-width apart.
2. Raise your heels off the ground until you are standing on your tiptoes.
3. Hold the position for 1-2 seconds and then slowly lower your heels back down to the starting position.

Reps: 3 sets of 15-20 repetitions

Step-ups

Target area: Quadriceps, hamstrings, glutes

Steps:

1. Stand in front of a step or bench.
2. Step up onto the step or bench with your right foot.
3. Push yourself up until your right leg is fully extended.
4. Step down with your right foot and repeat with your left leg.

Reps: 3 sets of 10-15 repetitions on each leg

Side leg raises

Target area: Outer thighs, glutes

Steps:

1. Lie on your right side with your right arm bent at the elbow and your right hand under your head.
2. Raise your left leg up until it is parallel to the ground.
3. Hold the position for 1-2 seconds and then slowly lower your leg back down to the starting position.

4. Repeat on the other side.

Reps: 3 sets of 10-15 repetitions on each leg

Deadlifts

Target area: Hamstrings, glutes, quadriceps, back

Steps:

1. Stand with your feet shoulder-width apart and a barbell in front of you.
2. Bend at the waist and grasp the barbell with an overhand grip, shoulder-width apart.
3. Keep your back straight and your core engaged as you lift the barbell up to your hips.
4. Slowly lower the barbell back down to the starting position.

Reps: 3 sets of 5-8 repetitions

Hip thrusts

Target area: Glutes, hamstrings, quadriceps

Steps:

1. Sit on the ground with your back against a bench and your feet flat on the floor.

2. Place a barbell across your hips.
3. Drive your hips up until your body forms a straight line from your shoulders to your knees.
4. Slowly lower your hips back down to the starting position.

Reps: 3 sets of 10-15 repetitions

Bulgarian split squats

Target area: Quadriceps, hamstrings, glutes

Steps:

1. Stand in front of a bench with your back to it and your right foot placed on the bench.
2. Hold a dumbbell in each hand at your sides.
3. Lower your body down until your left thigh is parallel to the ground.
4. Drive through your left heel to push yourself back up to the starting position.
5. Repeat on the other side.

Reps: 3 sets of 10-15 repetitions on each leg

Glute bridges

Target area: Glutes, hamstrings

Steps:

1. Lie on your back with your knees bent and your feet flat on the floor.
2. Place your arms at your sides.
3. Raise your hips up off the ground until your body forms a straight line from your shoulders to your knees.
4. Slowly lower your hips back down to the starting position.

Reps: 3 sets of 10-15 repetitions

Lunges with rotation

Target area: Quadriceps, hamstrings, glutes, obliques

Steps:

1. Stand with your feet shoulder-width apart.
2. Step forward with your right leg and lower your body down until both knees are bent at a 90-degree angle.
3. Rotate your torso to the right, bringing your right elbow towards your left knee.
4. Push back up to the starting position and repeat with your left leg.

Reps: 3 sets of 10-15 repetitions on each leg

CHAPTER 5

Stretching Exercises

Stretching is an important part of any workout routine, but it is especially important for seniors. Enhancing flexibility, range of motion, and balance can be achieved by stretching. Additionally, it might lessen aches and pains in the muscles and enhance blood flow.

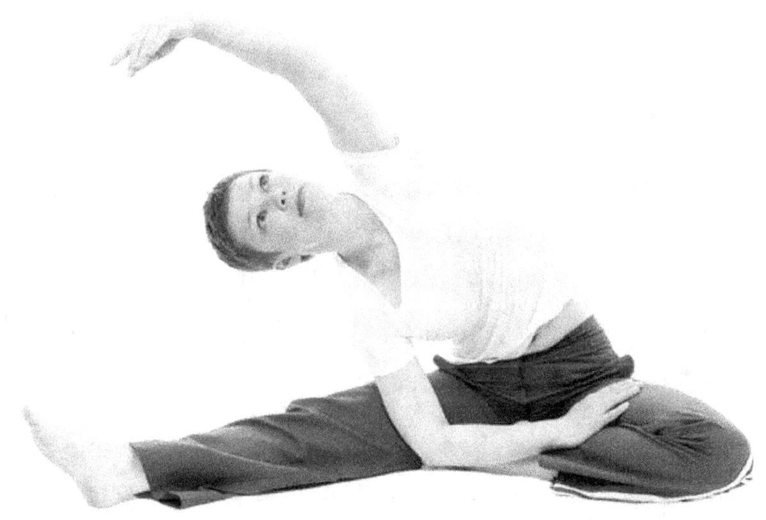

Simple stretches that seniors can do:

Neck stretches

Neck tilt: Tilt your head to the right side and bring your right ear towards your right shoulder. After holding the stretch for 10 to 15 seconds, switch to the other side.

Chin tuck: Tuck your chin towards your chest and hold the stretch for 10-15 seconds.

Neck rotation: Slowly rotate your head in a clockwise direction and then in a counter clockwise direction. Repeat 10 times in each direction.

Shoulder stretches

Arm circles: Stretch your arms forth and inward in little circles. Gradually increase the size of the circles and the speed at which you are moving your arms.

Shoulder rolls: Roll your shoulders forward and backward 10 times in each direction.

Arm across the chest: Place your right hand on your left shoulder and raise your right arm across your chest. Gently pull your right arm towards your chest and hold the stretch for 10-15 seconds. Repeat on the other side.

Back stretches

Knee to chest: While lying on your back, place your feet flat on the ground and bend your knees. With both hands, raise one knee to your chest and hold it there. Stretch your knee gently toward your chest, holding the position for 10 to 15 seconds. Continue on the opposite side.

Cat-cow: With your back flat, begin on your hands and knees. Arch your back and raise your gaze as you inhale. Turn your back and tuck your chin in toward your chest as you release the breath. Do these ten times.

Child's pose: Place your knees hip-width apart on the ground. Fold forward, putting your forehead on the floor while you sit back on your heels. With your hands facing down, extend your arms in front of you. Stretch for 10 to 15 seconds.

Hip stretches

Knee hug: Stand on one leg and bend your other leg, bringing your foot up to your buttock. Grab your foot with your hand and gently pull it towards your buttock. After holding the stretch for 10 to 15 seconds, switch to the other side.

Hip circles: Stand with your feet shoulder-width apart. Place your hands on your hips and make small circles with your hips in both directions. Gradually increase the size of the circles and the speed at which you are moving your hips.

Butterfly stretch: Sit on the ground with your knees bent and your feet flat on the floor. Bring your knees out to the sides and bring your feet together. Gently press your knees down towards the ground and hold the stretch for 10-15 seconds.

Leg stretches

Stretch your hamstrings by sitting on the floor and extending your legs in front of you. Maintaining an upright back, extend your hand toward your toes. Stretch for 10 to 15 seconds.

Stretch your quadriceps by placing your feet shoulder-width apart. Grab your foot with your hand while bending one leg behind you. Stretch your heel gently toward your buttocks, holding the position for 10 to 15 seconds. Continue on the opposite side.

To stretch your calves, face a wall and lay your hands shoulder-height on the wall. While keeping your rear heel on the ground, place one foot behind the other. Till your rear leg's calf begins to stretch, bend forward. After holding the stretch for 10 to 15 seconds, switch to the other side.

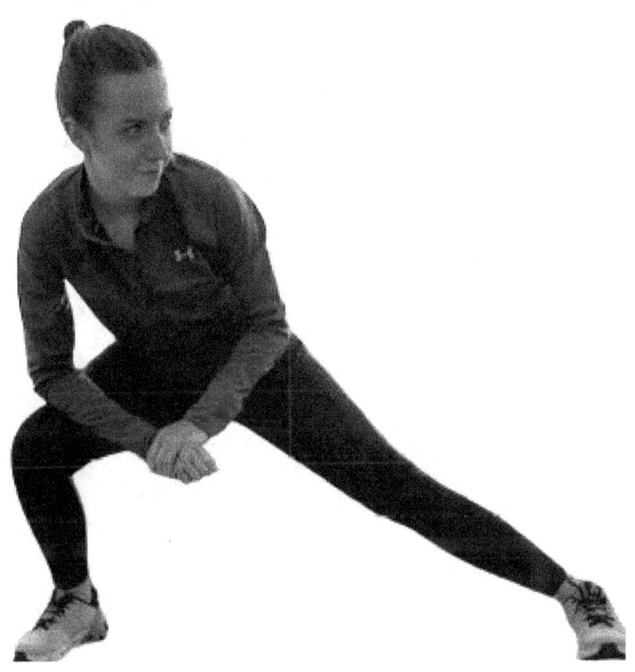

Chest stretches

- Stand in a doorway with your forearms placed against the doorframe at shoulder height.
- Until your chest starts to extend, lean forward.
- Hold the stretch for 10-15 seconds.

Triceps stretch

- Stand with your feet shoulder-width apart.
- Bend one arm behind your head and grab your elbow with your other hand.
- Gently pull your elbow towards your head until you feel a stretch in the back of your upper arm.
- Repeat on the opposite side after holding the stretch for 10 to 15 seconds.

CHAPTER 6

Beginner Bodyweight Workout For Seniors

Beginner bodyweight exercises are a good place to start if you're new to exercising or recuperating from an injury. This kind of exercise is easy on your joints and minimal impact.

Beginner Bodyweight Workout Sample

Warm-up.

- 5 minutes of mild exercise, such marching or walking in place
- 10 forward and backward arm circles
- 10 neck tilts to the right and left
- 10 shoulder rolls to both sides.

Work Out

Squats: 10 to 15 reps

Wall push-ups: 10 to 15 reps

Crunches: 10 to 15 reps

Leg raises: 10 to 15 reps

Plank: 30-60 seconds

Cool-down

- 5-minute mild cardio
- **10 hamstring stretches:** With your legs out in front of you, take a seat on the ground. Maintaining an upright back, extend your hand toward your toes. Stretch for 10 to 15 seconds.
- **10 quadriceps stretches:** Stand with your feet shoulder-width apart. Grab your foot with your hand while bending one leg behind you. Stretch your heel gently toward your buttocks, holding the position for ten to fifteen seconds. Continue on the opposite side.

Intermediate Bodyweight Workout Sample

You can go to an intermediate bodyweight workout if you feel comfortable with the beginner's routine. Despite being more strenuous, this type of exercise is still low-impact and nice to the joints.

Warm-up.

- 5 minutes of moderate cardio
- 10 forward and backward arm circles

- 10 forward and backward shoulder rolls
- 10 head tilts, both to the left and right

Work out

Squats: 15 to 20 reps

Knee push-ups: 15 to 20 reps

Cycle crunches: 15 to 20 reps

Leg raises: 15 to 20 reps

Side plank: every side for 30 to 60 seconds

Cool-down

- 5 minutes of moderate cardio
- 10 hamstring exercises
- 10 quadruple-stretches

Advanced Senior Bodyweight Exercise

A challenging and well-maintained bodyweight exercise is an option for advanced bodyweight training. This kind of exercise is quite demanding and calls for a lot of stamina and strength.

Warm-up.

- 5 minutes of moderate cardio
- 10 arm circles, two in each direction
- 10 shoulder rolls, one in each direction
- 10 head tilts, both to the left and right

Work out

Pistol squats: 10 to 15 reps per leg

Complete push-ups: 10 to 15 reps

Twisted leg raises: 10 to 15 reps on each side

Russian twists: perform each side 15–20 times.

Bird dogs: do 15–20 reps on each side.

Cool-down

- 5 minutes of moderate cardio
- 10 hamstring exercises
- 10 quadruple-stretches

Squats: If you have difficulty balancing, you can hold onto a chair or wall while squatting. You can begin with chair or half squats if you have knee problems.

Push-ups: If you are unable to do a full push-up, you can start with knee push-ups or wall push-ups.

Rows: If you have difficulty bending over, you can do seated rows.

Lunges: If you have difficulty balancing, you can hold onto a chair or wall while lunging. If you have knee pain, you can start with step-ups instead of lunges.

Plank: If you have difficulty holding a plank, you can start with your knees on the ground.

Modifications For Seniors With Specific Limitations

Arthritis: You might want to stay away from joint-stressing workouts if you have arthritis. Low-impact activities like walking and bicycling, as well as water aerobics and swimming, are beneficial forms of exercise for those with arthritis.

Osteoporosis: Exercises that strengthen your bones and enhance your balance are the things you should concentrate on if you have osteoporosis. Walking, jogging, and dancing are among excellent weight-bearing workouts for adults with osteoporosis. Exercises like planks and crunches that work your core muscles should also be incorporated.

Heart disease: It's crucial to see your doctor before beginning any new fitness regimen if you have heart problems. Your doctor can assist you in developing a program of safe and efficient exercise. For those with heart disease, walking, swimming, and biking are among beneficial forms of exercise. Additionally, you want to do upper body strengthening activities like bicep curls and rows.

CHAPTER 7

How to avoid injuries

- Prior to exercise, warm up. Warming up lowers your chance of injury and gets your body ready for exercise. Dynamic stretches and light cardio for five to ten minutes provide a fantastic warm-up.
- Take note of your body. The moment you experience any pain, cease the workout. Don't overwork yourself.
- Apply correct form. To prevent injuries, it's important to exercise with correct form. When working out, ask a certified personal trainer for help if you need it.
- You should begin your workouts slowly and gradually increase the length and intensity. Refrain from attempting to handle too much at once.
- Put on appropriate footwear and clothing. Put on comfortable, loose clothing that won't limit your mobility. Put on supportive and traction-rich shoes.

When To Stop Exercising

Signs you should stop exercising:

- Chest pain
- Shortness of breath
- Dizziness
- Light-headedness
- Nausea
- Severe pain
- Confusion

Stop exercising immediately and get help if you observe any of these symptoms.

Nutrition for seniors

Eating a healthy diet is important for everyone, but it is especially important for seniors. Seniors need to make sure that they are getting enough nutrients to support their active lifestyle.

Tips for eating a healthy diet as a senior:

- Eat a lot of vegetables, fruits, and entire grains. These foods are high in vitamins, minerals, and fiber.
- Select lean protein sources such as fish, chicken, legumes, and tofu.

- Reduce intake of unhealthy and saturated fats.
- Achieve enough vitamin D and calcium. The health of the bones depends on these nutrients.
- To keep hydrated, take lots of water throughout the day.

Staying Motivated to Exercise

- It can be difficult to stay motivated to exercise, especially as we age. Here are a few tips:
- Set achievable goals. Refrain from attempting to handle too much at once.
- Find a workout partner. Maintaining your motivation and accountability when working out with a friend or family member might assist.
- Include exercise in your daily regimen. Set aside time every day or every week to exercise.
- Look for things to do that you enjoy. If you don't enjoy your workouts, you are less likely to stick with them.
- Give yourself a reward for achieving your objectives. This might be anything from treating yourself to a special supper to purchasing a new clothing for your workout.

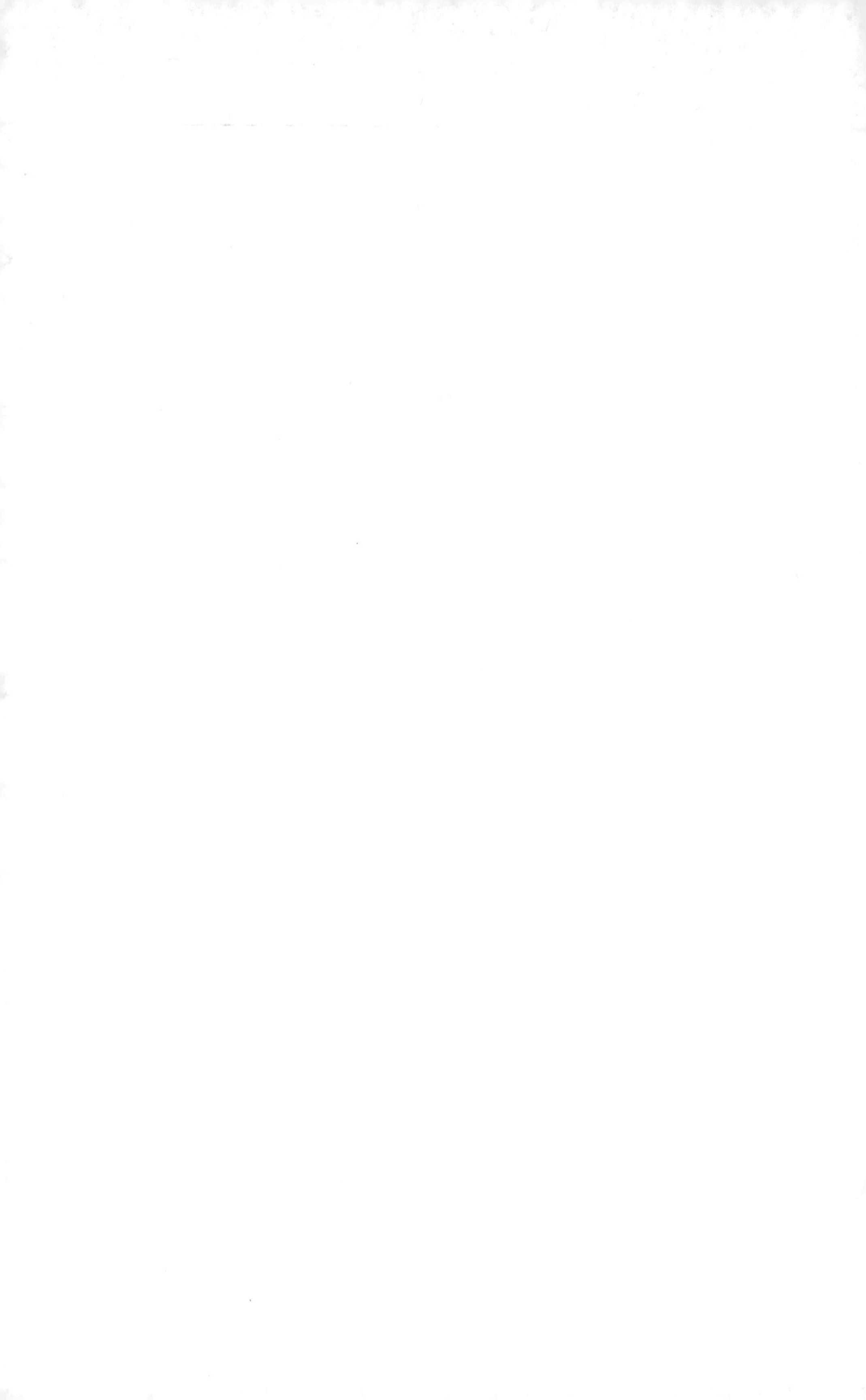